HEALING NATURE OF URINE THERAPY.

URINE THERAPY AND ITS TRADITIONAL USES.

A traditional therapy treatment for hair loss, Arthritis, Cancer, Migraines, dandruff, and application for teeth whitening and for skin also, for eradication of eczema, rashes and dry skin.

By

Charles Amelia.

Table of Contents

CHAPTER ONE.

WHAT IS URINE?

Urine is a clear, transparent liquid that is usually golden brown. The average urine output in 24 hours is 5-8 cups or 40-60 ounces. Chemically, urine is primarily an aqueous solution of salt, urea and uric acid. It typically contains approximately 960 parts of water to 40 parts of solids. Abnormally, it may contain sugar (as in diabetes), albumin (a protein, as in some forms of kidney disease), bile pigments (as in jaundice), or an abnormal amount of one or other of its normal components. Kidneys. produces urine by filtering waste products and excess water from the blood. The waste is called urea. Your blood carries it to your kidneys.

Urine is stored in a particular portion of the body and urinated out when the person feels like it. It swells round when full and shrinks when empty. A healthy body can hold up urine for as long as more than 3 hours.

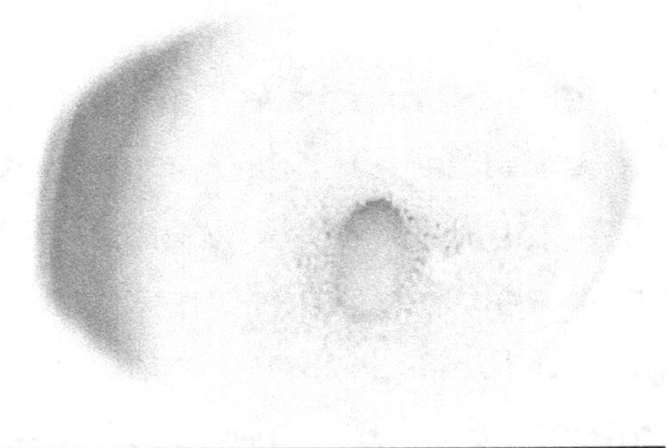

Urination.

Urination, is the emptying of urine from the bladder Nerve centres that focus on controlling urination are located in the spinal cord, brain stem and cerebral cortex (the outer substance of the upper part of the brain). Both voluntary and involuntary muscles are involved.

The bladder is a storage container for urine - a liquid that contains waste products that the body excretes and passes through the kidneys into the bloodstream. The main contracting muscle of the bladder is the detrusor. Urination involves either continuous or short alternating contractions of the detrusor and contraction of the urethral muscle, which is the tube to the bladder that removes urine from the body. In humans and most other animals, bladder emptying is affected by the amount of urine it contains. When 100 to 150 millimetres (3.5 to 5 ounces) of urine accumulates, the first urge to urinate occurs. The feeling of well-being increases when more urine accumulates, it becomes unpleasant when the volume of the bladder is 350-400 millimetres. Nerve impulses in the pelvic area transmit the sensation of bladder filling, painful swelling and the conscious need to urinate. A slowly filling bladder gradually adjusts to the pressure of the increased volume. Thus, a rapidly filling bladder stimulates urination faster than a slowly filling bladder. When the bladder walls can be felt.

There is enough pressure, the detrusor muscle contracts, the bladder neck and urethral opening relax, and the contents of the bladder are emptied. The bladder usually empties. Voluntary restriction of urination involves preventing the bladder from contracting, closing the urethral opening and contracting the abdominal muscles. The pelvic floor does the job of urine flow control. Lack of urinary control in young children is associated with nervous immaturity. Consequently, the degeneration or destruction of certain areas of the central nervous system leads to urinary incontinence, the cause of which is the so-called neurogenic bladder.

Such incontinence can be a droplet overflow from a permanently distended bladder or leakage from a contracted bladder with the outlet always open. If a full bladder does not empty, it is overinflated. Over time, bladder swelling can lead to bleeding, ulcers, and tearing of the bladder wall. Urinary obstruction can be caused by swelling of the prostate gland (a gland surrounding the urethra near the bladder in men), swelling of the urethral tissue surrounding its canal, fibrotic stress on the urethra, or contraction of the opening muscles. bladder and urethra.

Urine is usually held until bladder pressure overcomes the blockage. With moderate chronic abstinence and stress, the tone of the detrusor muscles increases and the force of contraction of the bladder increases. When overstretching occurs over a long period, the detrusor muscle produces small, rhythmic

contractions that cause urine to drip. As a result of constant stretching, the muscle can become paralyzed, and the emptying of urine occurs only as a result of overflow; this condition is often called passive incontinence. Under these conditions, urine can also leak back into the kidneys, mainly causing kidney failure.

However, urine is a liquid waste that is produced in the body and excreted from the body. Through the renal tubules, it is excreted into the bladder and excreted through the urethra. Although it is 91 to 96 per cent water, it contains many other components, both solid and liquid.

Urine is a liquid or semi-solid solution consisting of metabolic waste and some other, often toxic, substance that the excretory organs

remove from the circulatory fluids and carry them out of the body.

CHAPTER TWO.

HISTORY AND DISCOVERY OF URINE.

About 6,000 years ago, laboratory medicine began with uroscopy analysis of human urine, later called urinalysis. The word "uroscopy" comes from two Greek words: "ouron" means urine and "skopeo" means to look, weigh, examine, and check. Ancient doctors spoke of urine as a window into the body and its inner workings and described various diseases. For example, Hindu cultures recognized "a strain of sweetness; in certain people and in urine that attracted black ants. Hippocrates (460-355 BC) hypothesized that urine is a filtrate of body fluids from the blood filtered by the kidneys.

Findings have it that when bubbles appear in urine it's just mainly a sign of possible kidney infections or maybe a trace of fever. Galen used the term "diarrhoea" for urine and described excessive urination. Theophilus Protospatharius, a seventh-century physician who wrote the first manuscript focusing solely on urine, called "De Urinisandquot"; noted that heating urine precipitates proteins and documented proteinuria as a disease.

The 12th-century physician Ismail de Jurjani recognized that food and ageing change the composition of urine and was the first to recommend a 24-hour urine collection.

Corbeil was one of the first scientists in at early 12th century, when he distinguished urine as a phenomena analysis based on colours hence he then classified them accordingly. De Corbeil also introduced a "matula" glass vessel in which the doctor could judge colour, texture and clarity. In 1630, French astronomer and naturalist Nicolas Fabricius de Peiresc made the first microscopic description of uric crystals and quorum; a mass of rhombic bricks. Later, in the early to mid-1800s, English doctor Richard Bright pioneered the field of kidney research, which led to him being later recognized as the "Father of Nephrology."

These few examples illustrate how urinalysis was the first laboratory developed in history, how it has been used continuously for several thousand years, and how it remains an excellent and cost-effective way to obtain important information for diagnostic purposes.

Other urine finds show that 1,000 years later, the first primitive monocular and compound microscopes appeared in the Netherlands, and as the Enlightenment progressed, urine was studied along with many other objects and liquids. Crude early instruments did not allow for good exploration due to chromatic and linear/spherical blurring. only Lister in London in the 1820s and Chevalier and Amici in Paris avoided these problems by making and using sophisticated multiclass lenses, making the urine microscope a practical and clinically useful tool in the 1830s.

Clinical microscopy of urine was pioneered by Rayer and his students in Paris (especially Vigla) in the late 1830s and reached Great Britain and Germany in the 1840s, with urinary sediments and composition of urine mode and knowing cells present and the Golden Bird. Donné especially taught in Paris. After another 50 years, optical microscopy reached its peak, and the immersion technique achieved magnifications of more than 1,000 times without aberrations.

Urine sediment atlases have been published in all major European countries and the United States. Polarized light and phase contrast continued to be used in the study of urine after the 20th century, and in the early 20th century, photomicroscopy (which Donné and Daguerre had done 50 years earlier but was then ignored) became common in teaching and recording. In the 1940s, electron microscopy was introduced, followed by the detection of specific proteins and cells with immune fluorescent antibodies. All this was done using the portable method.

Machine-assisted observations began around 1980 and have dominated ever since.

CHAPTER THREE.

ANIMAL HABITAT AND TYPES OF URINE EXCRETED.

Water is one of the basics that help to determine other mixtures in urine. Freshwater animals usually excrete very dilute urine. Marine animals try to combat the loss of water in their salty environment by excreting concentrated urine; Some are actively developing methods to remove salts.

Land animals, depending on their habitat, usually retain water and excrete highly concentrated urine. In most mammals, including humans, urine formation begins in the nephrons of the kidney by filtering blood plasma into the nephron; As the fluid passes through the nephron tubule, water and useful plasma components such as amino acids, glucose, and other nutrients are reabsorbed into the bloodstream, leaving behind a concentrated waste solution called final urine or bladder urine.

In addition, all unusual substances that do not have a mechanism to be reabsorbed into the blood remain in the urine.

Degradation products of nucleic acids occur in most mammals such as allantoin and humans such as uric acid and in Dalmatian dogs for reproductive purposes, but insoluble uric acid The urine of birds and reptiles is a whitish aqueous suspension of crystals of uric acid, which is discharged into the sewer and mixed with faeces before the faeces are removed. Ground insect urine is solid and in some cases is stored as a pigment in the body instead of being eliminated. Amphibians and fish excrete aqueous solutions of urea; However, unlike mammals, their excretory organs do not reabsorb large amounts of water, so their urine remains liquid.

Some marine animals store large amounts of urea in their blood, which slows osmotic water loss. In small primitive animals (teleost fishes, echinoderms, coelenterates and unicellular animals), especially aquatic animals, the end product of amino acid metabolism is the highly toxic ammonium gas, which is collected and removed from the dilute aqueous solution. Many smaller animals do not develop an excretory system; each cell transports its wastes into the circulatory fluids and then the wastes are distributed to the surrounding environment.

URINE COMPOSITION.

Urine osmolarity is a way of estimating urine concentration and can vary between 50-1200 mOsmol/kg. on average, the solute in urine is about 1000 mmol/day and urine is excreted about 1.4 litres per day.

The amount of hydration and salt level makes up most urine composition. Carnivores have higher solutes because they get a lot of urea from their muscles, while vegetarians, who get most of their energy from carbohydrates, produce fewer solutes. Some solids dissolve in the urine, with a total of 24.8- 37.1 g of solutes.

In the urine./kg. Uric solids consist mainly of organic matter, mainly volatile solids. Urine contains large amounts of nitrogen, phosphorus and potassium. Urine has some organic acids in the presence is nitrogen and has a gulf of up to 50. This includes urea from protein metabolism, sodium and potassium, both of which come from food. Thus, the dry matter contains 14-18 per cent of nitrogen, 13 per cent of carbon and 3.7 per cent of potassium and phosphorus. Most of these substances are excreted from the body in urine.

Urine Calcium.

Calcium excretion is affected by protein intake, as described above, and sodium excretion is strongly affected. A low sodium diet therefore reduces calcium excretion and vice versa. A normal adult urine sample collected over 24 hours should yield a calcium concentration of 100 to 250 mg.

Nitrogen Excretion.

Nitrogen is excreted in the urine mainly as urea, on average about 11 g of nitrogen is excreted per day. It is most influenced by dietary protein intake, and the correlation between dietary protein and urinary nitrogen components is 0.91. About 80 per cent of the nitrogen in food is balanced by nitrogen compounds excreted in the urine. Urea concentration in urine varies between 9-23 g/l. Creatinine is another important urinary nitrogen compound, the amount of which depends on body weight muscle mass and age. Gender differences may correlate with these. The creatinine production of the body is on average about 1.6 g/day Nitrate is the third nitrogen compound in urine, the concentration of which increases when a person follows a protein-rich diet.

In addition to the protein in the diet, it causes changes in the nitrogen content of the urine. other minerals such as phosphorus and potassium. In addition, very low protein intake can affect calcium levels.

Kinds Of Urine.

The types of urine can be distinguished using the colour of urine at a given point in time.

Normal urine.

The colour of normal urine varies from clear to pale yellow. But some things can change the colour. For example, foods like beets, blackberries, and beans can make your urine pink or red. Some medications can give urine bright colours, such as orange or green-blue.

Unusual Or Abnormal Urine.

Colour can also be a sign of health problems. For example, some urinary tract infections can make urine milky white. Kidney stones, some cancers and other diseases sometimes make urine red because of blood. A quick check for various symptoms that indicate abnormal urine; The normal colour of urine varies. Fluids dilute the yellow pigments in the urine. Research has it that water intake has the capability of purifying the body's urine. If you drink less, the yellow colour becomes stronger. But urine can change colour much more than usual, including:

- Blue.
- Green.
- Orange.
- Dark brown.
- Cloud white.
- Red.

However, a visit to the doctor is necessary if there is blood in the urine. This is a common infection and other related diseases that may cause difficulty in urine passage. These problems often cause pain. Or even result in cancellation that may cause so bleeding in Dark or orange urine. This may be a sign that your liver is not working properly, especially if you also have pale stools and yellow skin and eyes.

Main causes: Urine discolouration is often caused by certain medications, foods, or foods. Sometimes it is due to health problems. Here are some unusual urine colours and the things that can cause them. Remember that colours may look slightly different to different people. For example, colour variations are one keynote.

<u>Pink And Red Urine.</u>

People feel that red urine is the cause of unhealthy in humans, but it is not so research has it that it is not a sign of major illness.

<u>Orange Urine</u>.

blood health problems that can cause blood in the urine include an enlarged prostate, noncancerous tumours, and kidney stones and cysts. Some cancers can also cause blood in the urine. Strenuous exercise, such as long-distance running, can also cause bleeding.

 Medications. A tuberculosis drug called rifampin (Rifadin, Rimactane) can turn urine red-orange. So can the urinary tract pain reliever phenazopyridine (Pyridium). Constipation medications containing senna can also cause this colour.

Foods. Beets, blackberries, and rhubarb can make your urine red or pink.

The cause of orange urine is as follows;

Medicines. Phenazopyridine and some constipation medications can turn urine orange. So can sulfasalazine (azulfidine), a medication that reduces swelling and irritation. Some cancer chemotherapy drugs can also turn urine orange.

• Vitamin: Certain vitamins, such as A and B-12, can turn urine orange or yellow-orange.

• Health problems. Orange urine can be a sign of liver or biliary tract problems, especially if you also have pale stools. Dehydration can also turn your urine orange.

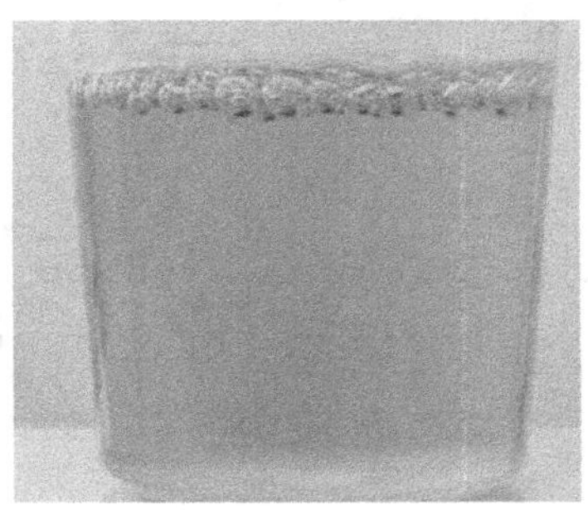

<u>A typical sample of orange urine.</u>

<u>Green And Blue Urine.</u>

The green and Blue Urine:

Dyes. Some bright food colourings can cause green urine. Dyes used in some kidney and bladder tests can turn the urine blue.

Medications. The antidepressant amitriptyline can turn your urine greenish-blue. So can a treatment for ulcers and reflux called cimetidine (Tagamet HB). A water pill called triamterene (Dyrenio) can also turn urine greenish blue.

 Urine can turn green because of indomethacin (Indocin, Tivorbex), used to treat pain and arthritis symptoms. Green urine can also be caused by propofol (Diprivan), a strong medicine that helps people sleep or relax before surgery.

Health problems. A rare condition called familial benign hypercalcemia can cause blue urine in children. Urinary tract infections caused by certain types of bacteria can cause green urine.

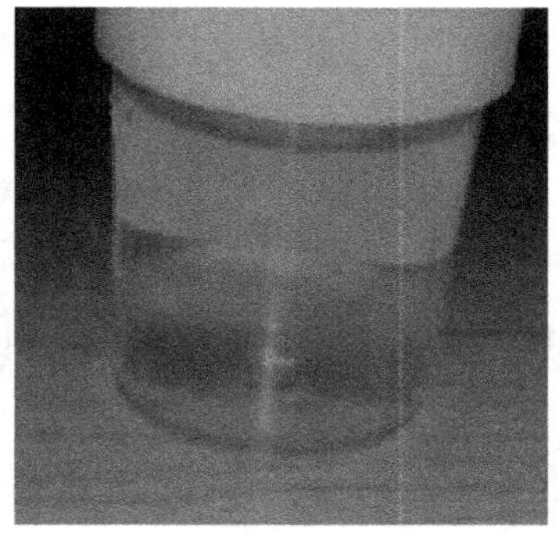

A Typical Green Urine Sample.

Cola-Coloured And Dark Brown Urine.

The major causes of brown urine are as follows:

• Food. Eating a lot of beans, rhubarb or aloe can cause dark brown urine.

• Medications. Some medications that darken urine are:

• quine which ends malaria.

• The antibiotics metronidazole (Flagyl, Metrocream, etc.) and nitrofurantoin (Furadantin, Macrobid, etc.).

• Constipation medications. include Sena (Senocot, Ex-Lax, etc.).

• Methocarbamol (Robaxin), a muscle relaxant.

• Anticonvulsant phenytoin (Dilantin, Phenytek).

• Cholesterol-lowering drugs called statins.

• Health problems. Some liver and kidney diseases and some urinary tract infections can make urine dark brown. So can bleeding inside the body, called haemorrhage. Some urine could be brown because of skin infections

• Extreme exercise. Muscle damage caused by heavy exercise can change the colour of urine tea or cola. Damage can cause kidney damage.

<u>Murky or cloudy urine.</u>

Urinary tract infections and kidney stones can make urine cloudy or cloudy.

Factors that pose a health risk and are capable of changing urine colour.

A change in urine colour that is not caused by food or medication may be due to a health problem. Some things that can put you at risk for health problems affect the colour of your urine.

• Family history. Maybe somehow hereditary

• Age. Older people are more likely to have bladder and kidney tumours, which can cause blood in the urine. Men over 50 sometimes have blood in the urine due to an enlarged prostate.

• Heavy exercise. Distance runners are most at risk. But anyone who exercises a lot can get blood in the urine.

CHAPTER FOUR.

URINARY OSMOLARITIES AND URINARY SYSTEM.

The osmolality of urine The osmolality of urine is the number of molecules (not affected by molecular size) per kilogram of water and must be measured with an osmometer.

It is used to assess renal concentrating ability and must be interpreted according to the patient's hydration and volume status. Urine-specific gravity is more commonly used to assess renal concentrating ability because it is easier to measure (with a portable refractometer). Specific gravity is the ratio of the density of a substance to the density of water, so it is affected by the number of molecules and their molecular weight. Urine Osmolality and Urine Osmolality Urine are usually linearly correlated. When urine contains many high molecular weight molecules, Urine Osmolality Urine overestimates the concentration of urine solute, while urine osmolality remains accurate. Some molecules that can interfere with USG are albumin, synthetic colloids and iohexal.

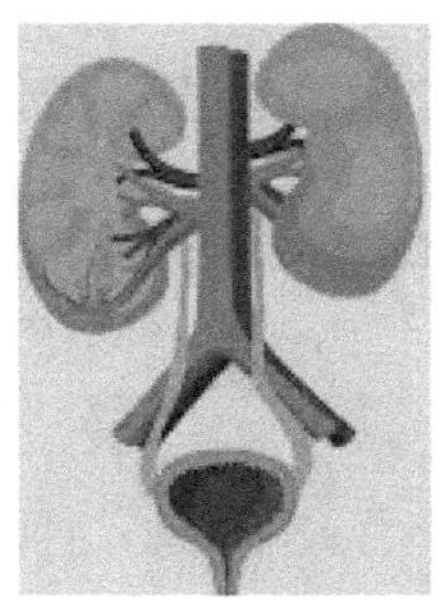

Urinary System

Interpretation of urine osmolality requires information about patient hydration and intravenous volume. This makes it possible to distinguish an appropriate renal physiological response from an abnormal physiological response.

Urinary Osmolarities Test.

How To Perform The Osmolality Test. A clean urine sample is required. The clean catch method is used to prevent bacteria from entering the urine sample from the penis or vagina. Urine is collected following medical advice whereby using a kit with clean solutions Follows the instructions exactly.

<u>Simple Way To Prepare For The Test.</u>

Your provider may advise you to limit your fluid intake for 12 to 14 hours before the test. Your provider will ask you to temporarily stop taking any medications that may affect the test results. Take your medication regularly until you talk to your healthcare provider. Other things may affect your test results.

received any type of anaesthesia for surgery;

• received an intravenous dye (contrast) for an imaging test such as a **CT** scan or MRI.

• used herbal or herbal medicines, especially Chinese herbs.

Possible Reaction To The Test.

The test involves normal urination. No discomfort.

Reasons For Osmolality Test Of Urine.

This test helps monitor your body's water balance and urine concentration. Urine osmolality is a more accurate measure of urine concentration than a urine-specific gravity test.

The Normal Outcome Of The Test.

Normal outcomes are as follows:

Hazardous specimen50-1200mOsm/kg(50-1200mmol/kg
12-14-hour fluid level: pli ol 850mOsmkg (850mmolkg)

Abnormal Outcome.

Normal values may vary slightly between laboratories. Talk to your provider about the meaning of certain test results.

A higher than normal Osmolality may indicate:

- Adrenal glands that do not produce enough hormones (Addison's disease or other types of adrenal insufficiency)
- Glucose (a type of sugar) in the urine
- Heart failure
- High sodium in the blood
- Loss of body fluids (dehydration)
- Narrowing of blood in the renal artery (renal artery stenosis)
- Shock
- Inappropriate ADH secretion syndrome (SIADH)

lower than normal osmolality may indicate:

- renal tubular cell damage (renal tubular necrosis)renal tubulitis (low nephritis).
- Kidney infection
- Low blood sodium
- Excessive
- fluid
- intake

<u>Formation And Creation Of Urine</u>.

The kidneys' job is to use urine to clean up the body. Urine formation has three main stages: glomerular filtration, reabsorption and excretion. These processes ensure that only waste and excess water leave the body.

Below are the stages of urine formation;

Glomerular filtration: Each kidney contains more than a million tiny structures called nephrons. The glomerulus is a network of capillaries surrounded by a cup-like structure, the glomerular capsule (or the capsule of Bowman). As blood flows through the glomerulus, blood pressure forces water and solutes from the capillaries through the filtering membrane into the capsule.

This glomerular filtration triggers the formation of urine. Filtration, within the glomerulus, blood pressure pushes fluid from the capillaries through a layer of specialized cells into the glomerular capsule. These components remain in the bloodstream. Filtrate (fluid that has passed through the membrane) flows from the glomerular capsule into the nephron.

Reabsorption: The glomerulus filters water and small solutes from the circulation. The resulting filtrate contains waste products and other substances necessary for the body: important ions, glucose, amino acids and smaller proteins. As the filtrate leaves the glomerulus, it flows into a channel in the nephron called the renal tubule.

The filtrate absorbed in the glomerulus flows through the renal tubule, where nutrients and water are reabsorbed into the capillaries. At the same time, residual and hydrogen ions move from the capillaries to the renal tubules. This process is called secretion. Urine flows from the nephron tubule into the collecting duct. It travels from the kidney through the renal pelvis into the urethra and down into the bladder. We have it that 95% of water is contained in urine. The nephrons of the kidney process blood and form urine through filtration, reabsorption and excretion. Urine consists of about 95% water as mentioned above and 5% waste products. Nitrogenous waste products excreted in the urine include urea, creatinine, ammonia and uric acid.

In this course of this book, we are going to also look at the urinary system in brief as part of the guild of formation of urine, which serves as a therapy which we will look at in other chapters of this book.

The Urinary System.

The urinary organ and its function is to filter blood and form urine as a waste by-product. The organs of the urinary tract include the kidneys, renal pelvis, ureters, bladder and urethra. In short, these organs that make up the urinary tract are explained and they work. Energy is been gotten from the food nutrients. When the body has absorbed the necessary parts of the food, the remains remain in the intestines and blood.

Kidney And Urinary Function.

The kidneys and urinary system help the body get rid of liquid waste products called urea and keep chemicals like potassium, sodium and water in balance. Protein and and vegetables after digestion are the main produce of urea. Urea is transported through the bloodstream to the kidneys, where it is excreted along with water and other waste products such as urine. Other important functions of the kidneys include regulating blood pressure and producing erythropoietin, which regulates the production of red blood cells in the bone marrow. The kidneys also regulate acid-base balance and retain fluid. The main functions of the two kidneys, a pair of purple-brown organs, are located under the ribs towards the middle of the back. Features include:

Balances body fluids.

Check red blood cell production.

Release hormones to regulate blood pressure. Etc.

In summary, kidneys remove urea from the blood through small filtering units called nephrons. Each nephron consists of small blood capillaries called glomeruli and a small tube called a renal tubule. Urea, along with water and other waste products, forms urine as it passes through the nephrons and renal tubules of the kidneys.

The Ureters.

These consist of two narrow tubes carrying urine from the kidneys to the bladder. The muscles in the walls of the ureter constantly tighten and relax, pushing urine away from the kidneys. If urine accumulates or is allowed to stand still, nephritis may occur. Every 10-15 seconds, a small amount of urine is emptied from the ureters into the bladder.

The Bladder.

The bladder has a triangular hollow organ shape and is located in the lower abdomen. It is held in place by ligaments attached to other organs and pelvic bones. Bladder walls are relaxed store urine and thus expand, the urethra passes out the urine and hence the bladder is flattened. The bladder of a typical healthy adult can hold up to two cups of urine for two to five hours.

The Two Sphincter Muscles.

These circular muscles prevent urine from leaking by closing tightly like a rubber band around the opening of the bladder.

Nerves In The Bladder.

People urinate on discretion as they don't need to be told to do so.

The urethra.

This tube allows urine to leave the body. The brain signals the bladder muscles to tighten, which forces urine out of the bladder. At the same time, the brain signals the sphincter muscles to relax so that urine can leave the bladder through the urethra. If all the signals come in the right order, urination happens normally.

Notable facts about urine are listed below;

- Normal healthy urine is a pale straw or clear yellow colour.
- Darker yellow or honey-coloured urine means you need more water.
- A darker brownish colour may indicate liver problems or severe dehydration.
- Pink or red urine can mean blood in the urine.

CHAPTER FIVE.

URINE THERAPY.

What is therapy?: The concept of therapy is simply referred to as the administration of treatments that help remedy health problems.

Urinary therapy can therefore be referred to as using urine for treatments and other health-related issues. Looking at how this therapy can be used by individuals we start with the collection of specimens and conditions for usage and look at some drawbacks and major therapy achievements.

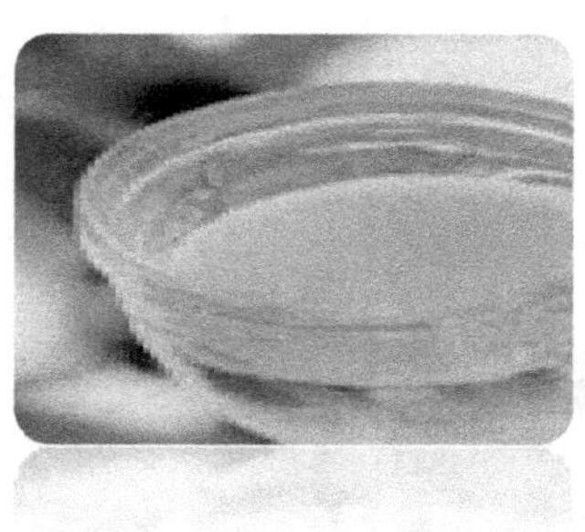

Urine Therapy.

<u>**Urinary Specimen Collections And Storage Mode.**</u>

Urine Specimens Procedures Collections: the urine specimen is about following some rules and other requirements and the quality control involved.

Rules: urinary specimens are carried to the laboratory with care diagnostic and treatment decisions based on the results. Clinical staff are responsible for patient instruction, collection and labelling of urine specimens, and timely transport of specimens to the laboratory.

Requirements of specimens: the requirements of the specimen which include special types and the mode of transportation of these specimens are elucidated below ;

<u>**Types of Specimen:**</u>

• **Random sample and 8-hour or first-morning sample:** A dried sample is generally more suitable for chemical and microscopic examination. A random sample can be taken indefinitely and is often more convenient for the patient. Random sampling is suitable for most screening purposes.

The patient should be advised to take the sample immediately after waking up from a night's sleep. Other 8-hour periods may be used for insomnia, night workers and certain children. Before lying down, the bladder is emptied and the sample is taken while standing so that the urine only reflects the lying position. Approximately **4444** overnight urines should be collected and combined with the first-morning urine sample.

• **2-3 hour postprandial and fasting samples:** Fasting differs from the first-morning sample in that it is the second void sample after fasting. After eating, the patient should be counselled immediately before eating a normal meal and tested 2 hours after eating.

• **All timed and catheterized samples:** To obtain an accurate timed sample, it is necessary to start and end the collection cycle with a blank sample. bladder The following 24-hour sampling guidelines can be applied to any scheduled collection (see test conditions for special preservatives required).Days 1-7: Patient voids and discards sample. During the next 24 hours, the patient collects all the urine.2.-7. day: the patient voids and adds this urine to the previously collected urine. A catheterized specimen is a specimen collected under sterile conditions by passing a hollow tube through the bladder.

• **Clean Collection, Pediatric and Suprapubic Specimens:** This specimen is a safer and less traumatic method of obtaining urine for bacterial cultures. It also provides a more representative and less contaminated sample for microscopic analysis than a random sample. The patient should have sufficient cleaning supplies and a sterile container. A "clean recovery" collection procedure. This may be a sterile specimen obtained by catheterization or suprapubic suction. A random sample can be taken by attaching a soft transparent plastic bag with glue to the general area of both boys and girls. Urine can be collected by inserting a needle from outside the bladder. At the same time, the suprapubic area is free of foreign contamination and can be used for cytological examination.

Transportation Specimens.

Urine should be delivered within 2 hours of collection or refrigerated and transported to the laboratory as soon as possible.

Possible ways to clean specimens are as follows:

- Single-use, clean, dry, tight container (sterile covered container is required for microbiological cultures).
- Screw on the sample tube and gloves are disposable
- Betadine suppositories (Hibiclens if you are allergic to betadine).
- Dry, clean gauze and the patient's bed base or urinal if the patient cannot go to the toilet.

<u>Quality Control And Required Calibration.</u>

As of now, no calibration is needed but for quality control to identify the patient, it is necessary to ask the conscious patient for his full name and date of birth. Check the identification strip if available.

<u>Collections procedures.</u>

Collection procedures are majorly done by preparing them before carrying out the procedures. For females let's see the procedures involved:

Female;

Before starting the procedure, wash your hands thoroughly and wear disposable gloves.

Use a betadine swab or Hibiclens to clean the perineal area.

Separate the labial folds and wipe the betadine swab or Hibiclens from one side to the back (front to back), then discard the swab or with the swab.

Using another betadine stick or Hibiclens, sweep one side from front to back and then discard.

Using a third Betadine swab or Hibiclens, wipe from centre to back and then discard.

Pat the dry periurethral area with clean dry gauze to remove excess Betadine, keeping the labia separated.

Male ;

In a similar way Before starting the procedure, wash your hands thoroughly and wear disposable gloves.

If the patient is uncircumcised, pull back the foreskin (foreskin) of the penis to clean it and hold it while urinating.

Clean the tip of the penis with a betadine swab or Hibiclens in a circular motion. Discard the stick or towel.

Urination must begin and the first part must be directed to the bed pot, urinal or toilet.

Once urine flow has begun, the urine sample container should be placed under when the patient collects the midstream (the "clean harvest" of the midstream) without contaminating the container.

Excess urine can seep into the bedpan, urinal or toilet.

Urinary should be covered properly. Transfer the urine to a specimen tube if tubes are used instead of urine containers for transport.

Attach the label to the tube or container and place the sample in the transport bag.

Remove gloves and wash hands.

Label the sample container with the date and time of collection and the initials of the collector (or sender) of the sample. Transport the specimen to the laboratory within 2444 hours of collection or refrigerate and transport it to the laboratory as soon as possible.

<u>**Procedure Drawbacks.**</u>

One major drawback is that the urine Osmolality cannot be collected with preservations.

CHAPTER SIX.

URINARY CULTURE AND URINARY TRACT

In the previous chapter, we have seen the composition, collection and storing of urine it is now best to look at urinary culture before moving further to its benefits and why people adopt it as a therapy.

A urine culture test checks for infectious bacteria (microorganisms) in the urine. Urine is your body's liquid waste (pee). Culture is the medical term for growing microorganisms such as bacteria and yeast in a laboratory environment.

Growth-promoting substances are added to the urine sample in the laboratory. If bacteria or yeast (fungus) are present, they begin to multiply. This growth indicates an infection in your urinary tract.

<u>**Why Urine Culture.**</u>

Healthcare providers order urine cultures for urinary tract infections (UTIs). A UTI can occur when bacteria enter the urethra, the tube that carries urine out of your body. Urinary tract infections usually start in the bladder (the organ that stores urine). They can spread to the kidneys (organs that produce urine) or to the prostate. A urine culture test also shows the bacteria or yeasts causing the infection, so the doctor can choose the most effective treatment and determine if the bacteria are resistant to antibiotics.

People Who Need A Urine Culture.

Your doctor may order a urine culture test if you develop frequent or difficult-to-treat urinary tract infections. Usually, only people who have symptoms of a urinary tract infection need a urine culture. Urinary tract infections can affect both sexes, but women are more affected than men.

Some frequent risk factors may include:

Problems emptying your bladder, especially if you use a urinary catheter to drain urine.

Frequent intercourse, especially with new persons or if you use spermicides.

Weakened immune system due to autoimmune diseases, organ transplant or cancer treatment.

Kidney stones and kidney disease

Diabetes

A Common Difference Between Urinalysis And Urine Culture.

Urinalysis and urine culture require a urine sample. A healthcare provider may first perform a urinalysis. This faster test checks the urine for red and white blood cells and bacteria that may indicate an infection. Urinalysis cannot detect certain bacteria that cause urinary tract infections. You will need a urine culture to get this information.

<u>**Some Common Infections That Urine Culture Can Easily Detect.**</u>

Below are some of the infections or diseases that a urine culture can detect during an exam. STLHs STDs: Healthcare providers sometimes use bacterial culture tests to diagnose STDs such as chlamydia and gonorrhoea. This test was not a urine culture test. Instead, healthcare providers grew (cultivated) cells from inside the urethra. Today, urinalysis can detect signs of these sexually transmitted diseases. However, to diagnose STDs, healthcare providers usually use more specific methods, such as testing fluid from the vagina or penis.

Escherichia coli E-spiral: A urine culture test can detect Escherichia coli (E. coli) bacteria. E. coli is the cause of most urinary tract infections. E. coli bacteria live in the digestive tract and are found in faeces. It is observed and proven that if stool is found it way into the vulva or penis is capable of causing the urethra to have bacteria hence, causes urinary tract infections. Your vulva (the outer part of your female genitalia where your vagina and urethra open) is near your anus. This is one of the reasons why women are prone to urinary tract infections. To prevent such infections, everyone should wipe from front to back after using the toilet, regardless of gender. Streptococcal infections: Group B streptococcus bacteria is a less common cause of urinary tract infections.

A urine culture can identify these bacteria living in the urinary tract and digestive tract. Group B strep is more likely to cause urinary tract infections in pregnant women. Treating the inflammation with antibiotics before delivery is crucial. The treatment prevents the transfer of bacteria from the pregnant woman to the newborn.

Urine culture preparation.

Do not urinate for at least one hour before giving the urine sample.

Drink at least 8 ounces of water 20 minutes before a sample to ensure there is enough urine for testing.

Take a urine sample first thing in the morning.

<u>Proceeds Or What Happens During Urine Culture</u>.

A urine culture requires a clean urine specimen. This term refers to a urine sample that is as free as possible of external contaminants, such as the common bacteria that live on your skin. You can have this sample delivered to your healthcare provider's office or a laboratory testing facility. In certain situations, you can take a urine sample at home.

A few steps are taken below:

- Keep both hands free from dirt
- Clean the opening of the urethra (vulva and vagina or head of the penis) with an antiseptic cloth.
- Pour a small amount of urine into the toilet, then stop mid-flow.
- Place a sterile cup under the vulva or penis before continuing to urinate Collect the prescribed amount of urine (usually 1-2 ounces) in the cup. Stop again mid-stream

(if possible) and keep the cup away until you finish urinating.

- Place the cup down, place the lid (if provided) and place it in the selected collection. Hands must remain clean.

Ways To Collect Urine Samples In Urine Culture.

For infants and young children and sick, hospitalized, or elderly adults, the healthcare provider may use one of the following methods for urine collection although some were mentioned in the previous chapter;

- **Catheterization:** A healthcare provider inserts a catheter (thin, flexible tube) through the urethra to access the bladder. Urine flows from the catheter into a sterile collection bag.

- **Aspiration:** A healthcare provider inserts a thin needle through the blister of skin on the undistracted abdomen to draw urine into a collection bag.

- **Urine bag (U-bag):** For babies and toddlers, you can attach a urine collection bag equipped with sticky glue directly to the penis or over the vulva. When your child has urinated, you empty their urine into a container with a lid. Keep the container refrigerated until you take it to the doctor's office or lab.

Duration to undergo urine culture.

Taking a clean urine sample only takes a few minutes. It shouldn't take very long to pee in a cup. Take the time to clean your vulva or penis before urinating to ensure clean urine. After the lab receives your urine sample, they grow the culture in an incubator for 24-48 hours. The incubator is set to the average human body temperature: 98.6 degrees Fahrenheit (37 degrees Celsius).

Risk Of Urine Culture.

Giving a urine sample using the clean capture method is very safe. There is a small risk of infection with the catheter or needle method.

A possible outcome of urine culture.

The lab may take up to three days to complete the test and return the results. Your healthcare provider will call you or ask you to come into the office to review the results.

- **Positive urine culture result:** If the urine culture test shows bacteria and you have symptoms of infection or bladder irritation, it means you have a urinary tract infection. The bacteria in the culture sample are subjected to an antibiotic sensitivity test in the laboratory. This test, also called an antibiotic susceptibility test, identifies the type of bacteria causing the infection and which antibiotics the bacteria are sensitive to, meaning which antibiotics will kill the bacteria. This information helps the doctor to choose the most effective antibiotic drug. Some antibiotics only work against certain bacteria. And some bacteria have antibiotic resistance. This means that the antibiotic can no longer prevent the growth of this type of bacteria. Infections that have higher resistivity are difficult to treat with antibiotics.

- **Negative urine culture result:** A negative or normal urine test result means that no bacteria or yeast were present in the urine sample. You don't have a UTI. The range of normal test results may vary depending on the laboratory performing the test. If you still have symptoms such as painful urination (dysuria) or blood in the urine (hematuria), your doctor may order imaging studies or other tests. In rare cases, these symptoms may indicate bladder cancer.

Urinary tract infection.

A urinary tract infection, commonly known as a UTI, is a very common type of urinary tract infection. It can affect any part of the urinary tract. Bacteria - especially E. coli

Symptoms include the need to urinate frequently, pain while urinating, and pain in the side or lower back. However, since urinary infection affects urinary tracts hence they are treated with some antibiotics as prescribed by healthcare providers.

This type of infection can affect you. Urethra (urethritis), kidneys (pyelonephritis), bladder (cystitis). Urine (pee) is a byproduct of the kidney's blood filtration system. Your kidneys make urine when they remove waste products and excess water from your blood. Normally, urine passes through the urinary tract without contamination. However, bacteria can invade your urinary system, which can cause urinary tract infections.

Urinary Tract:

The urinary tract forms and stores urine. That includes yours.

Kidneys: The kidneys are small bean-shaped organs at the back of the body, above the pelvis. Most persons have two kidneys. They filter water and waste products from your blood, which become your pee.

Ureters Your ureters are thin tubes that carry urine from your kidneys to your bladder.

Bladder: Your bladder is a balloon-like organ that stores urine before it leaves your body.

Urethra: a tube that is capable of carrying or allowing passage of urine from the body is known as the Urethra.

Urinary tract infections are very common, especially in women and people identified as female at birth (AFAB). About half of the people with AFAB will have a urinary tract infection at some point in their lives. Men and individuals male at birth (AMAB) can also get UTIs, as can children, although they only occur in 1-2% of children. Healthcare providers treat between 8 and 10 million people each year for urinary tract infections.

Symptoms Of Urinary Tract Infections:

Inflammation can cause the following problems.

- Pain in the side, stomach, pelvis or lower back.
- Cloudy, smelly pee.
- urinary incontinence.
- Frequent urination.
- Pain during urination (dysuria).

- Blood in the urine (hematuria).
- Pain in your penis.
- Feeling very tired (fatigue).

These are a few symptoms we can mention in this guild, however, there are many other symptoms not mentioned here which are out there some are still under study view.

Mode Of Transmission Of Urinary Tract Infections:

urinary tract infections are caused by bacteria. They usually enter through the urethra and can infect the bladder. The infection can also travel from the bladder through the ureter and eventually infect the kidneys.

Major Causes:

E. coli causes more than 90% of cystitis. E. coli is usually found in the intestines (colon). Anyone can get a UTI, but you are more likely to get a UTI if you have a vagina. This is because the AFAB of the human urethra is shorter and closer to the anus, where E. coli bacteria are common. You can get a UTI from your fingers. Your hands can collect bacteria and other microorganisms every time you touch a surface. You can accidentally release bacteria into the urethra by going to the bathroom or during sex, including masturbation or fingering. You must wash your hands before and after using the toilet or having sex.

Treatment Of Urinary Tract Infections.

Healthcare providers will help you out with your treatment.

Some other tests your doctor may perform are:

• **Urinalysis**: During this test, you pee into a special cup. The provider sends the sample to a lab, where technicians examine it for signs of urinary tract infection using several variables, including nitrites, leukocyte esterase, and white blood cells.

• **Urine culture:** You pee into a special cup and lab technicians check your sample for growth and bacteria. The right treatments the healthcare provider may need may result from Urine culture experiments. If your system is still resistant to treatment, another test method may be used:

• **Ultrasound:** look at your internal organs. For information's sake, it does not much discomfort

• **Computed tomography (CT):** A CT scan is another type of imaging. This is a type of X-ray that takes cross-sectional pictures of your body—like slices—and creates 3D pictures of the inside of your body. A CT scan is more accurate than an ordinary X-ray.

• **Cystoscopy:** In a cystoscopy, the inside of the bladder is viewed with a cystoscope through the urethra. A cystoscope is a thin instrument with a lens and light at the end. If you get frequent UTIs, your doctor may look for other health problems (such as diabetes or urinary tract infections) that may be contributing to your infections.

Management of the urinary tract infection by an individual.

The best thing to do with a urinary tract infection is to see a doctor. You need antibiotics to treat a urinary tract infection. Your provider will choose the antibiotic that works best against the bacteria responsible for your infection. If you have received a prescription for antibiotics, it is very important to follow the instructions for taking them. Remember to take the full course of antibiotics, even if your symptoms go away and you feel better. If you don't stop all medications, the infection may come back and be more difficult to treat. If you get a lot of UTIs, your provider may recommend antibiotics. Every day, every other day, after sex and at the first symptoms.

Some Medications Used In Treating Urinary Tract Infection.

Below are some medications that are used in treating urinary tract infections to get clean catch urine are as follows:

- Nitrofurantoin.
- Sulfonamides (sulfa drugs) such as sulfamethoxazole/trimethoprim.

Amoxicillin. Cephalosporins such as cephalexin.

- Doxycycline.
- Fosfomycin.

Quinolones such as ciprofloxacin or levofloxacin. If you get frequent UTIs, your doctor may give you a short-term, low-dose antibiotic to prevent the infection from recurring. Your provider may recommend this cautious approach to treating recurrent UTIs because your body may develop resistance to the antibiotic and you may develop other types of infections, including C. diff colitis. This practice is not very common.

Preventive Measures For Urinary Tract Infection.

• **Cleaning:** Maintaining good hygiene is one of the best ways to prevent urinary tract infections. Vaginal presence can have short urethra which has a better efficacy and it is easier for E. coli. To avoid this, always wipe from front to back after moving the bowels. During your period, it's also a good idea to regularly change your menstrual products, including pads and tampons. Smelling or pungent deodorant should be kept from the vagina.

• **Drink plenty of water:** Drinking extra fluids every day—especially water—can help flush bacteria from your urinary tract. Constant drinking of water a day is good for health.

• **Change your urinary habits:** peeing can play an important role in removing bacteria from the body. Your pee is waste, and every time you empty your bladder, you help remove waste from your body. Urinating regularly can reduce your risk of infection, especially if you have many UTIs. Sex can introduce bacteria into the urethra, and one thing that helps the body remove these bacteria is urinating during and after sex. If you can't urinate, wash the area with warm water.

• **Contraception:** Some people have a higher risk of getting a UTI if they use a diaphragm as birth control. Talk to your doctor about other birth control options.

• Using water as a lube during sex: If you use a lube during sex, make sure it's water-based. You should also avoid killing sperm if you have frequent UTIs.

• Wear different clothes: tight clothes can create a moist environment that encourages bacterial growth. You can try loose clothing and cotton underwear to prevent moisture from accumulating around the urethra. of.

CHAPTER SEVEN

SCHISTOSOMES.

In the course of this guild, we will look at some diseases that can be related to urine, it is very necessary to do this because the harvest of urine is clean, so these factors should not be ignored. We have seen an infection that can make urination almost impossible, so if the ducts are inflamed, then it is necessary to look at a urinary tract infection.

What is schistosomiasis: Schistosomiasis is an infection caused by trematodes. These schistosomes (also called platelets) are parasites belonging to the genus Schistosoma.

Parasites are creatures or organisms that live in or on another creature or organism (the host) and receive food from the host or that organism. It hurts the host. In schistosomiasis, snails are found in immune cells and then released into the water. If your skin comes into contact with contaminated water, the parasites can be transferred to you and live there for years.

The parasite, which infects humans after developing, has a kind of fork-shaped tip that allows it to penetrate the skin.

The three main types of schistosomiasis cause two main forms of the disease: urogenital schistosomiasis and intestinal schistosomiasis. It is estimated that more than 230 million people worldwide are infected with this type of schistosomiasis. Anyone can become infected with these parasites by swimming or bathing in contaminated water. Parasites are found in freshwater lakes, rivers and ponds.

Symptoms Of Schistosomiasis.

Many people have no symptoms of schistosomiasis. Early signs and symptoms (those that appear within a few days of infection) may include itching and a rash. Later symptoms (occurring within 30 to 60 days of infection) may include.

Blood in the urine (pee), also called hematuria.

Blood in the stool (faeces), also called hematochezia.

- Fever
- Difficulty or pain during urination (dysuria).
- Enlarged liver
- Miscarriage

Chronic (long-term) schistosomiasis can increase the chance of scarring of the liver or bladder. In rare cases, you may have eggs in your brain or spinal cord. If this is true, you may have seizures, paralysis, or spina bifida.

Schistosomiasis is caused by a parasite that lives in certain snails in freshwater areas. The parasitic form emerging from the snail penetrates the human skin with a bifurcated head. Infected people excrete egg-contaminated urine and faeces into water-containing snails. The eggs are transferred to the snails and the cycle continues. Infected children and adults become infected again and again.

However, people do not infect each other. If you have schistosomiasis, you cannot pass it on to another person. Scientists are working to find a way to control the disease. Some efforts focus on vaccine development and others on snail control.

Diagnosis Of Schistosomiasis.

Eggs are sometimes found in urine or faeces, but often a blood test is needed. All of them are examined under a microscope.

Management Of Schistosomiasis.

Schistosomiasis is treated with the prescription drug praziquantel (Biltricide).

The drug, which comes in pill form, belongs to a class of drugs called anthelmintics. This type of medicine kills worms. It is usually taken throughout the day as either one large dose or three smaller doses throughout the day. Before taking any medication, you should tell your doctor what other medications and supplements you are taking and what allergies you have. You should also ask if you can eat grapefruit or drink grapefruit juice while taking this medication.

Some Preventive Measures.

There are things you should not do in the fresh pond, lake or river water in areas known to harbour snails and parasites that cause schistosomiasis.

Don't assume water is safe just because people say so. In places where the parasite is known, it is best not to take any chances.

Not every water is fit for drinking, This doesn't mean you can get parasites by drinking the water, but they can get to the skin around your mouth.

Don't drink, swim, fish in this water

If you get wet clean up with a towel as soon as possible.

A look at what ways it affects urine and the concept of it.

Urinary Schistosomiasis.

It is caused by an intravenous infection caused by Schistosoma crematorium parasites. The adult worms usually migrate to the masses of veins in the human bladder and secrete eggs, which are excreted in the urine of the infected person. Chronic infection can cause serious illness and long-term complications when the eggs attach to human tissues, causing inflammation and fibrosis. Chronic infection can also increase the risk of liver fibrosis or bladder cancer. Because schistosomiasis causes blood in the urine, it is important to understand, that this disease is extremely dangerous and must be avoided or treated immediately after exposure. This has now led us to take a closer look at what bloody urine, also known as hematuria, means.

The Concept Of Blood Urine (Hematuria):

Seeing blood in your urine can be scary, also called hematuria. In many cases, the cause is harmless. Any time there is a blood spot in the urine is a symptom of serious illness. If you see blood, it is called hematuria. Blood that cannot be seen with the naked eye is called microscopic hematuria. It is such a small amount that it can only be seen under a microscope when the urine is examined in the laboratory. In any case, it is important to find out the cause of the bleeding.

Symptoms Hematuria:

Blood in the urine can be pink, red or cola-coloured. Red blood cells change the colour of urine. It only takes a small amount of blood to turn urine red. Bleeding is often painless. However, if blood clots appear in your urine, it can be painful. See your doctor whenever you see blood in your urine. Red blood cells are not always the cause of red urine. Some medications can make urine red, such as phenazopyridine, which relieves urinary symptoms. Certain foods, such as beets and rhubarb, can also turn your urine red. It can be difficult to tell if a change in urine colour is due to blood. That's why it's always better to get yourself checked. This condition occurs when the kidneys or other parts of the urinary tract allow blood cells to leak into the urine. This leak can be caused by a variety of problems, including.

Urinary tract infections (UTIs): They occur when bacteria enter the tube through which urine leaves the body, ie. In the urethra, the bacteria then multiply in the bladder. Urinary tract infections can cause bleeding, which turns urine red, pink, or brown. If you have a urinary tract infection, you may also have a strong need to urinate that lasts a long time. You may experience pain and burning when you urinate. Your urine may also have a very strong odour.

Kidney infection: This type of urinary tract infection is also called pyelonephritis. Infections can also occur when bacteria enter the kidneys through the tubes that connect the kidneys to the bladder, called the ureters. Kidney infections can cause the same urinary tract infections as other urinary tract infections. But they are more likely to cause fever and pain in the back, side or groin.

Bladder or kidney stones: Minerals in the urine can form crystals on the walls of the kidneys or bladder. Over time, the crystals can turn into small, hard stones. Stones are often painless. But they can cause a lot of damage if they cause a blockage or leave the body with urine. Bladder or kidney stones can cause blood in the urine that is visible to the naked eye, as well as bleeding that can only be detected in a laboratory.

Enlarged prostate: It often grows in middle age. It then presses the urethra and partially blocks the flow of urine. An enlarged prostate can cause difficulty urinating, an urgent or constant need to urinate, or blood in the urine. Inflammation of the prostate, called prostatitis, can cause the same symptoms.

Kidney disease: Blood in the urine, which can only be seen in a laboratory, is a common symptom of a kidney disease called glomerulonephritis. In connection with this disease, the small filters of the kidneys, which remove waste products from the blood, become inflamed. Glomerulonephritis can be part of a disease that affects the whole body, such as diabetes.

Cancer: Blood in urine visible to the naked eye can be a sign of advanced kidney, bladder or prostate cancer. These cancers may not cause symptoms earlier when treatment can work better.

Hereditary diseases: A genetic condition that affects red blood cells called sickle cell anaemia can cause blood in the urine. Blood cells may be visible or too small. Alport syndrome, which damages the small blood vessels in the kidneys, can also cause blood in the urine.

Kidney damage: A stroke or other kidney injury from an accident or contact sport can cause blood in the urine.

Medicatio: Penicillin Medicines that thin the blood.

clotting is also related to urine.

Hard training: You may have blood in your urine after playing contact sports such as football. It may be related to bladder damage caused by concussion. Blood in the urine can also occur in long-distance sports such as marathon running, but it is not as clear why. It may be related to damage to the bladder or other non-traumatic causes. If heavy exercise causes blood in the urine, it may go away on its own within a week.

Urine may contain some blood that may not be visible to the naked eye so for a clean catch however rigorous tests need to be carried out even before it can be used as a therapy.

CHAPTER EIGHT.

URINE THERAPY AND USES OF URINE.

How it works and other reasons:

Several possible explanations for how and why urine therapy works have been presented in this guide. These should not be seen as separate detail talks, but these multiple factors together give urine therapy its extraordinary effectiveness. Here are ten futures about the effectiveness of automatic urine therapy.

- Nutrient Absorption and Recycling
- Hormone Absorption
- Enzyme Absorption
- Urea Absorption
- Immunological Activity
- Bactericidal and Antiviral Activity
- Detoxification
- Diuretic Activity
- Psychological Activity.

This guide will provide more explanation on this future or hypothesis:

Absorption and recycling of nutrients: by drinking urine or rubbing it on the skin, many vitamins, amino acids, salts, hormones, etc. readily available in urine can be reabsorbed and recycled as nutrients. This is especially important during illness when diseased body tissue enters the blood and therefore must be removed. In the filtering process, the kidneys must break down this tissue into raw materials, which the body can then reuse to build new tissue. During the disease, the composition of urine changes, because some important substances do not reach their destination. And then they are filtered through the kidneys. A good example of this is a blockage in the liver, which can lead to hepatitis (inflammation of the liver). When the liver is blocked, the bile produced by the liver does not reach the intestines, but seeps into the blood and then ends up in the urine, causing weakness and nausea. The lack of bile in the digestive tract limits the digestion of fats and proteins.

Absorption of hormones: many hormones end up in the urine. The basis of this hypothesis is that we can bring them back into the body by drinking or rubbing with urine. Since proteins are damaged by gastrointestinal acids, pepsins and enzymes, the hormones reabsorbed from the urine when administered orally are mainly small, non-proteinaceous (protein complexes). Sex hormones, adrenal hormones and thyroid hormones are almost certainly reabsorbed, the effect of which remains to be studied. Applying urine externally to the skin allows the hormones to be absorbed back into the body without being destroyed. Urinary tract massage is therefore an important addition to urinary therapy because urine is absorbed directly into the tissues. Reabsorption can be necessary in two ways. First, certain hormones have very specific effects on the healing process. For example, corticosteroids secreted by the adrenal cortex prevent infections and have a positive effect on the treatment of allergies such as asthma and hay fever, skin diseases such as eczema and psoriasis, and inflammatory diseases such as rheumatism.

Hormone therapy is very effective in treating all of these conditions, but the role of these hormones in treatment has not yet been proven. Second, reabsorption can be a way for the body to conserve energy. general Taking hormones again allows the body to recycle at least some of them, so that energy does not have to be used to make new hormones. Hormones are very powerful molecules that require a lot of energy to produce. Once done, they are capable of completely changing the balance. bodily processes, personality, emotions and state of mind, even if only a few molecules are released. So even the slightest reabsorption of hormones can have a powerful effect on health and energy levels. Vice contains melatonin, a hormone released by the pineal gland that has a calming effect. The concentration of this hormone is higher in the first urine sample early in the morning. Melatonin also has powerful anti-cancer and anti-ageing effects. It is entirely possible that the ancient sages were well aware of the hormonal effects of urine. They argue that if a person cannot urinate, same-sex urine is acceptable, but not opposite-sex urine. Although cultural and social factors may have influenced this rule, the fact is that female urine contains significantly more female hormones, such as estrogen. . . if consumed by men for a long time, it can have a feminizing effect. The opposite happens with a woman who swallows a man's urine. Some recommend using the first urine after intercourse. During sexual stimulation, the higher endocrine glands release certain hormones that have a rejuvenating and rejuvenating effect on the body. Women and men are not left out.

Enzyme Absorption: Based on studies with the urokinase enzyme, positive results can be expected from the action of urinary enzymes. healthy". Urokinase found in human urine causes blood vessels to dilate and is similar to nitroglycerin in its ability to increase blood flow from the coronary artery to the heart muscle. Urokinase is extracted from urine and is available on the market as a lifesaver. There are many other active enzymes in urine, but more detailed information is not yet available.

Urea Absorption: Apart from water, the main component of urine is urea, which is the end product of modified proteins. A person excretes an average of 25-30 grams of urea per day. We come into contact with urea at an early age, i.e. as a fetus in the womb. The level of urea in the amniotic fluid, which consists mainly of fetal urine, doubles during the last two months of pregnancy. Before birth, we drink about half a litre of this liquid a day. The fetus also inhales it and it is essential for proper lung development. Scars disappear after fetal surgery due to the healing power of urea in the amniotic fluid in the womb.

According to scientists, 25% of an adult's urea reaches the intestine, where intestinal bacteria break it down into ammonia. Some of this ammonia reaches the liver, where some of it is converted to urea

the bladder is such a powerful anti-cancer drug. However, bladder cancer is a relatively rare form of cancer and usually only occurs in those who work with certain toxic chemicals, possibly interfering with or altering the effects of urea. Further research is needed on this topic. Urea also plays a very important role in the external distribution of urine, as it helps transport hormones through the skin. The enzymatic action of the digestive system destroys many hormones when urine is administered orally. In addition, administration through the skin ensures the absorption of hormones in the body slowly and in specific areas, which significantly increases its effectiveness. Urea can moisturize the skin and regulate its condition and structure, which is one of the reasons, why it is processed in many skin creams. Some pharmaceutical companies use horse urine to make urea, and in fact, there are many horses in the factory for this very purpose. Urea is an oxidizing agent that ensures that degradative proteins (proteins in the wound or inflammation) are broken down. It dissolves fats and other natural body secretions. Urea is even more effective when heated. Because of its strong antibacterial nature, urine inhibits the growth of tuberculosis bacilli.

The bactericidal or bactericidal activity of urine increases as the pH decreases. Urea and ammonia, which are close relatives, play an important role here. When complex polymers come into contact with urea, they change or break down into monomers that the body can tolerate.

Immunological Activity: Urine is not toxic, although some residues may be present in small amounts in urine, especially when a person is ill. When these triggering substances enter the body, the body's defence mechanisms (immune system) are activated. Unwanted waste that passes along with urine is likely the same as infection processes, balancing the entire system against other external attacks, meanwhile, how urine therapy is useful in the treatment of allergies. Similar process. occurs when a person is vaccinated against a certain disease, where a small amount of toxic substances is injected into the healthy body. This stimulates the immune system to produce antibodies (and thus protect the body) and can be called a homoeopathic or isopathic effect.

Reintroducing small amounts of bacteria or parasites in the urine can stimulate IgE production. IgA (an antiviral substance that prevents microorganisms from attaching to the mucous membrane) also plays a role in this. IgA is found in mucous membranes and body secretions, and thus also in urine. Treatment of the urinary tract increases the production of IgA, which may explain why this therapy has a positive effect on urinary tract and kidney infections, while other treatments do not provide much help. Several studies show that, for example, antibodies against Salmonella diphtheria, polio and HIV can be found in urine.

Bactericidal and Antiviral Activity: Although it is still not completely clear why urine has bactericidal and antiseptic effects, it is known that urea plays an important role. Ammonia and salt also have a similar cleaning effect. In addition to killing bacteria, urine also inhibits or destroys various viruses and fungi. Scientific studies have shown that both urea and ammonia have strong antiviral effects. Applying urine to a fresh cut or scrape prevents infection and keeps files away (important in hot climates).

Although urine does not completely prevent the growth of bacteria in the urethra (infections often occur), it has a strong antiseptic effect when used externally.

Herz also successfully treated urinary tract infections with urine therapy. Positive results may be due to the immune system stimulating the effect of ingested urine. As mentioned above, in this case, IgA is produced in larger quantities.

Detoxification therapy: Drinking salt water is an important therapeutic remedy during certain (fasting) treatments. Saltwater is also often used in yoga to thoroughly cleanse the body from the inside and relieve ailments such as asthma, stomach ulcers, indigestion and constipation. Drinking urine, which is also a salty substance, has the same effect.

This may be an important reason for the success of this therapeutic drug. Saline solutions remove old mucus stuck in mucous membranes. When someone drinks a saline solution, some of the salt goes into the body, where it dissolves excess mucus in the lungs and other organs. In addition to Imab urine, the excess water has become too watery due to the disease. Like a saline solution, urine also has a laxative effect and is recommended to relieve constipation. Soolejuha iräuskedes sölläb Sool ice kainen and draws water in the intestine, which facilitates the bowel. According to the theory, drinking urine, for example, drinking urine, drinking salt water, increases metabolism. It removes excess sugar from the blood and absorbs toxic substances from the cells. Thus, urine therapy is a good cleansing technology. These substances probably have a strong effect on mucous membranes and body cells to clap with saliva, which usually helps to clean wounds; Urine has the same effect. Saltwater is less effective than urine

Diuretic Actioins: In this phenomenon, urine therapy ensures that the kidneys work well and helps fast stimulate the body to produce more urine. Metabolic products made of proteins, such as urea, nitrogen and ammonia, are excreted from the body in urine as soon as there is an excess in the body. When drinking urine, more of these substances enter the body than usual. The body reacts by washing them away with water and other substances. When urine is ingested, the body is stimulated not only to excrete some of these metabolic products at an accelerated rate but also to convert some of them into useful substances. A previously mentioned example of this is urea, which is converted to glutamine by ammonia. For example, with gout, the body releases uric acid into the joints. The effect of flow and cleansing is especially felt during fasting. When you urinate for the first time while fasting, the urine is often thick and strong-tasting, especially if you have a fever or are otherwise ill. However, after drinking this initial amount, the second stream of urine will be thinner, even if no additional water has been drunk. Constant recycling of urine will produce large amounts of clear, foul-tasting urine over time. According to this hypothesis, this ultimately leads to stimulated and purified kidneys and purified blood circulation. At the same time, the intestines, skin and exhalation process will probably completely take over unusable metabolic products. Transmutation theory Transmutation theory needs a new holistic paradigm based more on dynamics than energies. Recent research shows a shift from reductionism to holism. Urine can be thought to contain an accurate holographic image of body fluids and tissues. Biofeedback of this holographic information through re-ingestion of urine can inform the energy system in a way that helps restore the disturbed balance.

Psychological Activity: The initial shock of drinking urine can fundamentally challenge previously accepted ideas, releasing pent-up energy that can be used to strengthen the body and fight disease. According to researchers, the maximum acceptable placebo effect is 30%. However, a much higher percentage of people achieve positive results with urine therapy, which is remarkable because many people are often sceptical at first due to an aversion to urine and use urine therapy as a last resort. The latter means that urine as a holographic substance can affect all levels of being, from the physical through the emotional and electromagnetic fields of the mind to the finer genetic vibration information of the soul.

Urine has so many uses which can serve as a therapy for users, proven or not for specific purposes it has uses below are some uses and applications of urine and how it serves as a therapy.

Uses Of Urine Therapy.

Urine Application To The Skin.

urine therapy is simply the use of urine for medical purposes instead of regular medications prescribed by a doctor or healthcare provider. some people have previously claimed to apply it to the skin to treat certain problems, but this has not been medically proven. Today's beauty trends. We're Not Sure About Urine Skin Therapy Yes, we're talking about the little ones. In your face, literally. Adjacent skin therapy involves collecting your urine and spreading it over your face and body. This is not a joke. The first slice or sample of the day is the best because it contains "supernutrients and antibodies." However, we are still quite shocked by the whole concept. Urine skin care can help with acne, eczema, rashes and dry skin, so any skin type just needs a little bit of it. It is said to increase the flexibility and elasticity of our skin. Healthy skin normally contains 28 micrograms of urea per square centimetre, while dehydrated skin has 50% less and anyone with a rash has 80% less.

Urine Application To Remedy Hair Loss.

The benefits of urine for hair are backed by science. Scalp massage has been shown to rejuvenate follicles and treat hair loss by stimulating growth. It is an antiseptic that can help treat several scalp problems such as infections, itching and dandruff. The Romans knew this and filled huge cisterns with the sewage used to clean Togo because it could dissolve fat.

The topical application of urine is believed to combat hair loss and stimulate hair growth. First, collect the urine let the first drops flow without interruption and collect the rest in a cup. Whether you want fresh or expired urine, both can be used for application. Before applying, gently heat the urine for 2-3 minutes, let it cool completely and remove the crust that forms on the surface. Dip a cotton ball in the liquid, part the hair and apply the urine to the scalp and hair roots. Massage lightly into the scalp and leave for 30 minutes to an hour before rinsing with lukewarm water.

Keynote:

Although urine is a simple "blood product", its use can be a big deal. But if you pay for it.

If you're trying urine therapy, eat plenty of fresh fruits and vegetables instead of animal proteins.

Eat well but the food should have less weight. Avoid using too many spices in your food.

Drink plenty of water throughout the day because you don't want highly concentrated urine for this purpose.

Many claim that this remedy has helped them successfully fight hair loss. After all, it is a natural medicine without side effects and worth trying.

Urine Is Used As Teeth Whitening.

Its natural whitening effect meant that urine was also used as toothpaste or mouthwash to give them a bright smile - only the very brave get by these days, rather than undergo expensive teeth whitening.

Cow Urine Therapy

Animal urine also has some uses we will look at cow urine and its effective applications: Cow urine is an effective disinfectant. Therefore, it is effectively used to treat dandruff, scalp infections and many other infectious diseases. A well-known and undoubtful feature of cow urine is the fact that it has an antioxidant effect. It is a very powerful healing element in cow urine that repairs damaged and dysfunctional tissues. Healing with cow urine brings good health and balances the doshas.

Today, people are constantly improving their health thanks to our care and treatment. This increases the continuity of their daily life.

Combined with cow urine, some medicines can act as adjunctive therapy to reduce the side effects of high doses, mental stress, radiation and chemotherapy. We teach people to live peaceful and stress-free lives with terminal illnesses, if any. Thousands of people have lived healthy lives after consulting us and it is a huge achievement for us to give them the life they dream of.

cow urine has a special status, often considered useful for the most troublesome diseases, such as hair loss. Our years of careful work show that almost all complications of hair loss disappear when using our herbs. Sufferers report that they notice a great change in their psychosocial results, that they control and balance hormonal and chemical changes in the body, slow down the rate of pigmentation and skin irritation. It also improves the patient's immune system, which works favourably in other complications of hair loss.

Urine also has benefits for plants. It also serves as fertilizer. In this guide, we will also look at how urine can serve as fertilizer.

Uses Of Urine As Fertilizer And Its Application.

Urine is rich in nitrogen and phosphorus, as well as many secondary and trace elements that plants need for growth. It's a balanced, plant-based diet that comes directly from your body for free every day. Currently, water treatment systems and infrastructure across the country and the world are under increased stress due to unpredictable weather conditions and ageing components. As a result, human waste can contaminate rivers, lakes and groundwater if these systems fail. So when we use peas in our garden, we not only give our plants what they need, but we also divert the waste stream. Abundant field trials with herbs over many years have shown that urine and chemicals are equally effective.

fertilized plots of land; both significantly higher than unfertilized blocks. Forage quality remained high and one farmer managed to achieve a stable second mowing of hay with urine for fertiliser. In the past, the harvest was not enough to harvest again. Compared to outdoor conditions, urine is a much higher quality fertilizer. This may seem surprising because we are so used to using different fertilizers in the garden.

Human urine contains more than 80% nitrogen and more than 65% phosphorus that we excrete every day. Pee contains more of the good stuff that plants need than faeces. Urine also does not contain pathogens and bacteria like faeces and is relatively easy to disinfect if necessary.

Urine can carry some viruses and bacteria, so if you use it on vegetables, share it with people outside your home, says World Health. The organization recommends disinfecting it. This means it must be stored in an airtight container for at least 6 months or pasteurized by heating at 160-180°F for 30 minutes before use. If you only use urine from your own home for vegetables eaten by households, there is no need for disinfection.

The amount needed to fertilize grain is enough to grow wheat to make bread every year. So, depending on the size of your garden, you may not need other sources of nitrogen and phosphorus. But remember that urine does not replace the important role of compost, organic matter and mineral additives such as kelp when needed. Nitrogen dissolves well in water and anything that is not taken up by green growing plants is washed away. Use urine only on green and growing plants (not on germinating seeds, small seedlings or plants that have reached the fruiting stage).

The best way to apply urine is as a mulch directly on moist soil. If your soil is dry, you can dilute the urine with water (we usually use a ratio of 1:1) or with water immediately after application. Never spray urine directly on the leaves or stems of the plant, but pour it into the soil about 4 inches from the base of the plant.

The Intake And Primary Use Of Urine By Individuals As Medicine.

Oral consumption of freshly voided morning urine has been recommended for many ailments such as viral or bacterial infections. Symptoms reported in the first few days of oral urine include nausea, vomiting, headache, palpitations, diarrhoea, or fever. Several substances found in urine, such as urea, uric acid, cytokines, hormones or urokinase, are thought to be important when administered orally.

Topical urine treatments include cleansing, packing local tumours, bathing the entire body or feet with urine, using urine as an eye wash, ear or nose drops, and using urine to clean a wound. Some practices have found that applying urine has been used to enhance healing. for some infections and diseases or to reduce their effects due to religious beliefs or traditional way of life, it is good in this guide to give the facts and what you think urine management has done so far in treating these infections.

The guide also explains the common disadvantages associated with the use of urine therapy, as below are some of the conditions that urine therapy can treat:

- Asthma
- Allergies
- Arthritis
- Cancer
- Indigestion
- Infertility
- Migraines

We will then look at some of these conditions urine therapy can be used as a way to reduce its effects and total cure.

Cancer Treatment Using Urine.

Camel urine has traditionally been used to treat many human ailments and has the most beneficial effects compared to the urine of other animals. However, scientific review of the protective effects of camel urine on cancer, platelets, stomach and liver is limited. Karmeli Uritsa had a significant cytotoxic effect in mouse bone marrow cells at a concentration of at least 50%; A marked decrease in the ratio of polychromatic erythrocytes (PCE) to normochromatic erythrocytes (NCE) indicates cytotoxicity in Carmel's urine. Al-Yousef et al. In 2012, CU was found to have anticancer properties in various cancer cells. Ten types of cancer cells were treated with 16 mg/ml CU. Again, complementary and alternative medicine is traditionally widely used in Saudi Arabia.

One of the most common practices is the use of camel urine alone or mixed with camel milk to treat cancer, often supported by religious beliefs. Another practice is that if you drink urine and then wash your eyes and sinuses (with a Neti pot), use it. brush your teeth and apply it to your skin.

The idea of this treatment as an anti-cancer treatment probably stems from the fact that tumour proteins are found in the urine of cancer patients. If urine enters the digestive tract and other parts of the body, it is a misunderstanding. that the body begins to produce antibodies against tumour proteins (antigens) in an attempt to destroy cancer. While it is true that urine can contain tumour antigens, there is no evidence that drinking, massaging with urine, bathing or any other use of urine stimulates antibody production or fights cancer in any way. The amounts of substances found in urine, including tumour antigens, are usually small compared to the amounts already present in the blood and elsewhere in the body.

The bottom line is that drinking your urine is probably not harmful, but it has no known medical benefits.

Arthritis Using Urine As A Treatment.

Cow urine is believed to have various medicinal properties. It is often used in traditional and religious ways or is believed to cure various ailments, including arthritis. Cow urine is said to contain hormones, enzymes and minerals that can help reduce inflammation and pain associated with arthritis. After the cow's urine method of treatment, some herbs rejuvenate the arthritic body lesions (Vata, Bile and Phlegm) if they can be proportionate. Some medicines contain many useful substances for their treatment. It improves the body's metabolismCow urine has a special status, which is often considered useful in the treatment of terrible diseases such as arthritis. In most cases, arthritis disappears with the use of traditional herbs and cow urine.

Patients report that they notice great relief from joint and muscle pain, knee swelling, stiffness, redness and fatigue, that they control and balance hormonal and chemical changes in the body, and that they improve the patient's immune system, which also works favourably in the body other forms of arthritis. The general concept of using urine to treat arthritis has not yet been clinically proven, but it has been a traditional practice to treat this arthritis, and all of the above findings are based on research and have not yet been proven or approved by the World Health Organization. organization (WHO).

migraine using urine as a treatment.

Urine like that of cow can be used based on the traditional ways and believe in treating migraines with other herbs in a mixture. cow urine can act as an additional medicine to limit many reactions caused by high-dose use, mental stress, radiation and severe headaches.

A few mentioned above in this guide have explained that people use urine as therapy in treating some diseases based on tradition but not clinically approved this practice is on for most parts of the world to date. This guide does not produce state or country details that practice such but brings to your notice that such practice is very much alive, we have seen some ailments and how urine is used coupled with some medication or herbs as practised in treating these diseases, same way urine is used to treat asthma, allergies, indigestion and infertility with other medication added in the process, note that some make use of other animal urine other than using human urine.

CHAPTER NINE.

RECYCLING OF URINE.

RECYCLING URINE TO FERTILIZER PRODUCTION:

Human urine is rich in nitrogen and phosphorus. Plants need these nutrients to grow. Now Finnish scientists have come up with a new way to separate them from human urine. And they say that this process can make a profit. Pee is mostly water. The rest is waste, which leaves the body with urine. One of these waste products is excess nitrogen. Nitrogen in urine is mostly a chemical known as urea (Yu-REE-uh). Urine also removes excess phosphorus from the body.

Both nitrogen and phosphorus are nutrients that plants need to grow. But spraying urine directly onto fields is impractical. Untreated urine can also contain harmful bacteria that can make people sick. So scientists are looking for ways to process pee into a safe and usable plant fertilizer. Much of this African country and other poor countries have few water treatment systems. Untreated human waste can pollute waterways and cause disease. Notes Pradhan, "Worldwide, sewage is a very big problem." Methods to make fertilizers from urine already existed.

One process produces magnesium ammonium phosphate crystals. Its common name is struvite. This can be useful for farmers when they need to fertilize food crops with phosphorus and nitrogen. But farmers don't always need both. The first step in their new process is to add calcium hydroxide to the urine. Calcium hydroxide is a basic chemical, also known as a base. This raises the pH of the urine above 12. (The alkaline range of the pH scale goes from just over 7, which is neutral, to a high of 14.) A high pH kills all bacteria and sterilizes urine. Calcium hydroxide also reacts chemically with urine. This pulls the phosphorus out of the mixture in the form of calcium phosphate.

This chemical can be sold as a phosphorus-rich fertilizer. Ammonia gas, which contains a lot of nitrogen, is also produced during the reaction.

The new process directs the gas into another chemical reaction vessel. It contains sulfuric acid. Here, ammonia reacts with acid to form ammonium sulfate. This is a common nitrogen fertilizer. Scientists continue to work with these fertilizers to see if they contain potentially harmful contaminants. For example, high levels of some metals can cause health risks.

How To Recycle Urine Safely:

Urine most times is collected from the comfort zone of the house, collected urine can also be useful in the household. To use the nutrients that come with the urine, it can be recycled as agricultural fertilizer. Previous studies have shown that urine can be effectively used as an alternative to traditional fertilizer. The urine produced by humans worldwide contains enough nutrients to fertilize three-quarters of the food we eat.

Below is what you need to do.

- Something to collect urine - urinal, urine drainage toilet or clean bucket.

Get a small container

Alkaline material with a pH of at least 10, such as ash from wood burning or slaked lime from limestone conversion. Choose something that can be applied in agriculture.

A fan that you attach to the tank and connect to electricity or a battery.

- Fill the tank with an alkaline material. If you choose slaked lime (about USD 1/kg), add about 3 kg per month for a family of four.
- Using a pipe the separation toilet is connected to a tank.
- To remove humid air from the bathroom, attach an exhaust fan to the tank.
- Urinate in the toilet as usual or pour the newly collected urine into a container immediately.
- Put on the fan
- This process is repeated monthly
- At the end of the month, you collect a dry powder that contains about 9% nitrogen,

1% phosphorus and 4% potassium. Store it for a few days at a temperature above 20 ° C. This ensures that the product is safe to handle and use in the home according to the guidelines of the World Health Organization.

Use it as fertilizer according to the needs of your plants.

Start the process again by replacing the tank with a fresh alkaline material.

Risk Of Drinking Urine.

Urine is a powerful combination of salts and chemicals that your body is trying to get rid of. These chemicals can cause serious health problems when used. Urine also has health benefits that other foods and drinks do not. These drugs leave your body in a state very similar to when they entered your body; they are not broken. Drugs that are excreted in this way include penicillin and all water-soluble drugs. Drinking urine containing these drugs carries them into the body. If these are medications you already take, increase the dose more than prescribed. If you drink someone else's urine, you could be taking medication that was not prescribed for you. This can cause dangerous reactions and serious health problems. contrary to popular myth. It contains bacteria like all other bodily secretions. Depending on the method of urine collection, it may also contain bacteria from the genital tract of the urine source. Drinking any type of urine can cause serious health problems if it is not sterilized separately. Your urinary system works specifically to remove toxic substances from your body. When dangerous substances begin to accumulate in the body, urine is one of the most important ways to eliminate them. Everything your kidneys filter out of your body is stored in your urine to be eliminated. When you drink urine, you are ingesting toxins that your body was specifically designed to eliminate. This can cause kidney damage or disease because these organs have to work harder to deal with the increased concentration of toxic substances.

Limited Or Overlooked Risk In Using Urine.

Urea, a compound found in urine, can be helpful when applied topically. The toxic effect of drinking urine does not manifest itself when it is applied to the skin. Synthetic urea is even found in skin care products. When it comes to hydration, water, electrolyte drinks, and most other beverages are probably safer than urine. Swallowing urine is of no use; all other drinks probably have fewer health risks. Although small amounts of urine probably won't hurt, they won't help either.

THE END

www.ingramcontent.com/pod-product-compliance
Lightning Source LLC
Chambersburg PA
CBHW071041250726
48653CB00005B/1935